My Diabetic Smoothie

Don't Miss This Delicious Collection of Diabetic Smoothies to Boost Your Energy

Valerie Blanchard

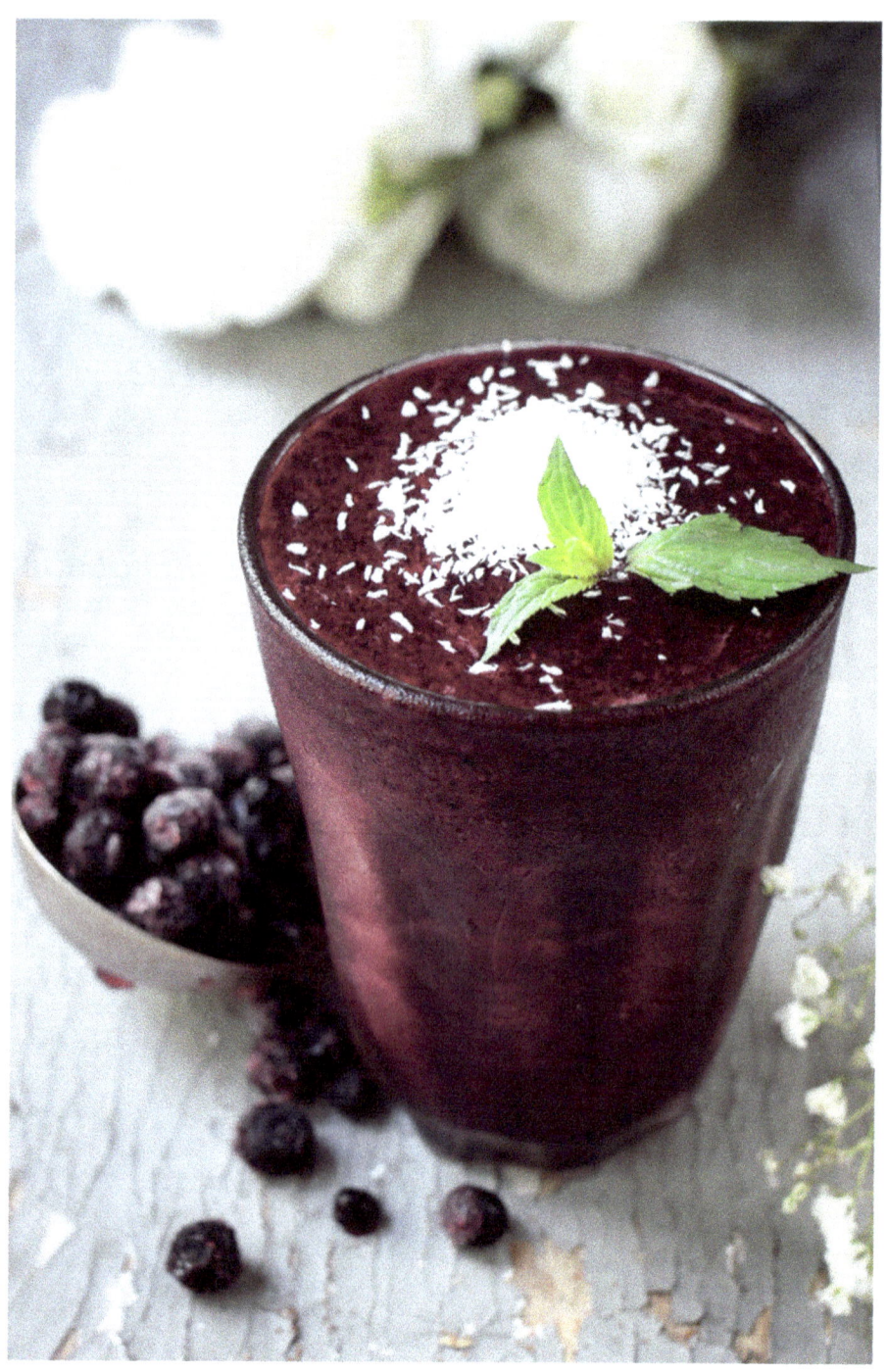

© Copyright 2021 - All rights reserved.

The content contained within this book may not be reproduced, duplicated or transmitted without direct written permission from the author or the publisher.
Under no circumstances will any blame or legal responsibility be held against the publisher, or author, for any damages, reparation, or monetary loss due to the information contained within this book. Either directly or indirectly.

Legal Notice:
This book is copyright protected. This book is only for personal use. You cannot amend, distribute, sell, use, quote or paraphrase any part, or the content within this book, without the consent of the author or publisher.

Disclaimer Notice:
Please note the information contained within this document is for educational and entertainment purposes only. All effort has been executed to present accurate, up to date, and reliable, complete information. No warranties of any kind are declared or implied. Readers acknowledge that the author is not engaging in the rendering of legal, financial, medical or professional advice. The content within this book has been derived from various sources. Please consult a licensed professional before attempting any techniques outlined in this book.

By reading this document, the reader agrees that under no circumstances is the author responsible for any losses, direct or indirect, which are incurred as a result of the use of information contained within this document, including, but not limited to, — errors, omissions, or inaccuracies.

Table of Contents

Banana & Strawberry Smoothie 7

Cantaloupe & Papaya Smoothie 9

Watermelon & Cantaloupe Smoothie 11

Raspberry and Peanut Butter Smoothie 12

Strawberry, Kale and Ginger Smoothie 13

Berry Mint Smoothie 15

Greenie Smoothie 17

Coconut Spinach Smoothie 19

Oats Coffee Smoothie 21

Veggie Smoothie 23

Avocado Smoothie 25

Orange Carrot Smoothie 28

Blackberry Smoothie 30

Key Lime Pie Smoothie 32

Cinnamon Roll Smoothie 34

Strawberry Cheesecake Smoothie 36

Peanut Butter Banana Smoothie 38

Avocado Turmeric Smoothie 40

Lemon Blueberry Smoothie 42

Matcha Green Smoothie 44

Blueberry Smoothie 46

Beet & Strawberry Smoothie 48

Kiwi Smoothie 50

Pineapple & Carrot Smoothie 52

Oats & Orange Smoothie 54

Pumpkin Smoothie 56

Red Veggie & Fruit Smoothie 59

Kale Smoothie 61

GREEN TOFU SMOOTHIE	63
GRAPE & SWISS CHARD SMOOTHIE	65
MATCHA SMOOTHIE	67
BANANA SMOOTHIE	69
STRAWBERRY SMOOTHIE	71
RASPBERRY & TOFU SMOOTHIE	73
MANGO SMOOTHIE	75
PINEAPPLE SMOOTHIE	77
KALE & PINEAPPLE SMOOTHIE	80
GREEN VEGGIES SMOOTHIE	82
AVOCADO & SPINACH SMOOTHIE	84
RAISINS – PLUME SMOOTHIE (RPS)	86
NORI CLOVE SMOOTHIES (NCS)	88
BRAZIL LETTUCE SMOOTHIES (BLS)	90
APPLE – BANANA SMOOTHIE (ABS)	92
GINGER – PEAR SMOOTHIE (GPS)	95
CANTALOUPE – AMARANTH SMOOTHIE (CAS)	97
GARBANZO SQUASH SMOOTHIE (GSS)	99
STRAWBERRY – ORANGE SMOOTHIES (SOS)	101
TAMARIND – PEAR SMOOTHIE (TPS)	103
CURRANT ELDERBERRY SMOOTHIE (CES)	105
SWEET DREAM STRAWBERRY SMOOTHIE	107

Banana & Strawberry Smoothie

Preparation Time: 7 minutes

Cooking Time: 0 minute

Serving: 2

Ingredients:

- 1 banana, sliced
- 4 cups fresh strawberries, sliced
- 1 cup ice cubes
- 6 oz. yogurt
- 1 kiwi fruit, sliced

Directions:

1. Add banana, strawberries, ice cubes and yogurt in a blender.
2. Blend until smooth.
3. Garnish with kiwi fruit slices and serve.

Nutrition: 54 Calories; 11.8g Carbohydrate; 1.7g Protein

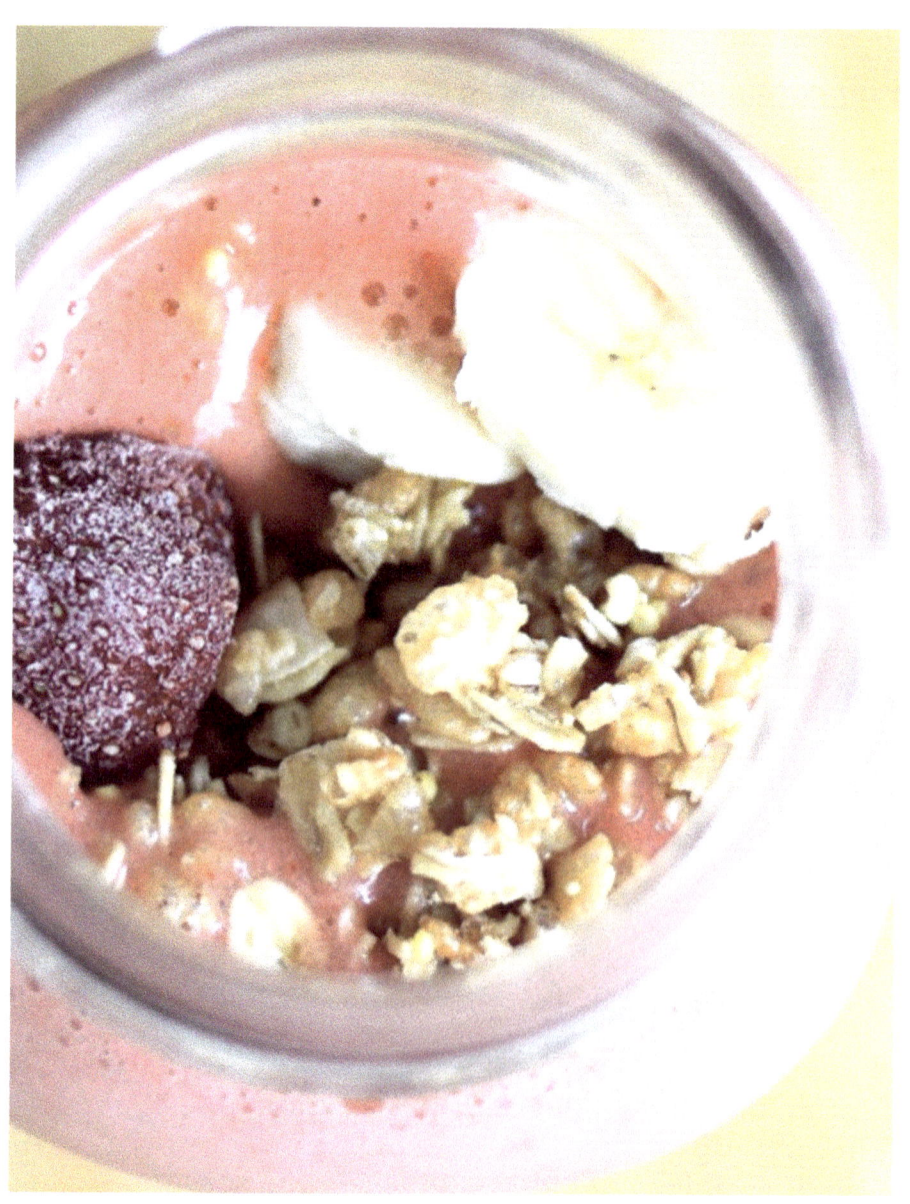

Cantaloupe & Papaya Smoothie

Preparation Time: 9 minutes

Cooking Time: 0 minute

Serving: 2

Ingredients:

- ¾ cup low-fat milk
- ½ cup papaya, chopped
- ½ cup cantaloupe, chopped
- ½ cup mango, cubed
- 4 ice cubes
- Lime zest

Directions:

1. Pour milk into a blender.
2. Add the chopped fruits and ice cubes.
3. Blend until smooth.
4. Garnish with lime zest and serve.

Nutrition: 207 Calories; 18.4g Carbohydrate; 7.7g Protein

Watermelon & Cantaloupe Smoothie

Preparation Time: 10 minutes

Cooking Time: 0 minute

Serving : 2

Ingredients:

- 2 cups watermelon, sliced
- 1 cup cantaloupe, sliced
- ½ cup nonfat yogurt
- ¼ cup orange juice

Directions:

1. Add all the **Ingredients** to a blender.
2. Blend until creamy and smooth.
3. Chill before serving.

Nutrition: 114 Calories; 13g Carbohydrate; 4.8g Protein

Raspberry and Peanut Butter Smoothie

Preparation Time: 10 minutes

Cooking Time*: 0 minute*

Serving*: 2*

Ingredients:

- Peanut butter, smooth and natural [2 tbsp]
- Skim milk [2 tbsp]
- Raspberries, fresh [1 or 1 ½ cups]
- Ice cubes [1 cup]
- Stevia [2 tsp]

Directions:

1. Situate all the **Ingredients** in your blender. Set the mixer to puree. Serve.

Nutrition: 170 Calories; 8.6g Fat; 20g Carbohydrate

Strawberry, Kale and Ginger Smoothie

Preparation Time: 13 minutes

Cooking Time: 0 minute

Serving: 2

Ingredients:

- Curly kale leaves, fresh and large with stems removed [6 pcs]
- Grated ginger, raw and peeled [2 tsp]
- Water, cold [½ cup]
- Lime juice [3 tbsp]
- Honey [2 tsp]
- Strawberries, fresh and trimmed [1 or 1 ½ cups]
- Ice cubes [1 cup]

Directions:

1. Position all the **Ingredients** in your blender. Set to puree. Serve.

Nutrition: 205 Calories; 2.9g Fat; 42.4g Carbohydrates

Berry Mint Smoothie

Preparation Time: *5 Minutes*

Cooking Time: 5 Minutes

Servings: *2*

Ingredients:

- 1 tbsp. Low-carb Sweetener of your choice
- 1 cup Kefir or Low Fat-Yoghurt
- 2 tbsp. Mint
- ¼ cup Orange
- 1 cup Mixed Berries

Directions:

1. Place all of the **Ingredients** in a high-speed blender and then blend it until smooth.
2. Transfer the smoothie to a **Serving** glass and enjoy it.

Nutrition: Calories: 137Kcal; Carbohydrates: 11g; Proteins: 6g; Fat: 1g; Sodium: 64mg

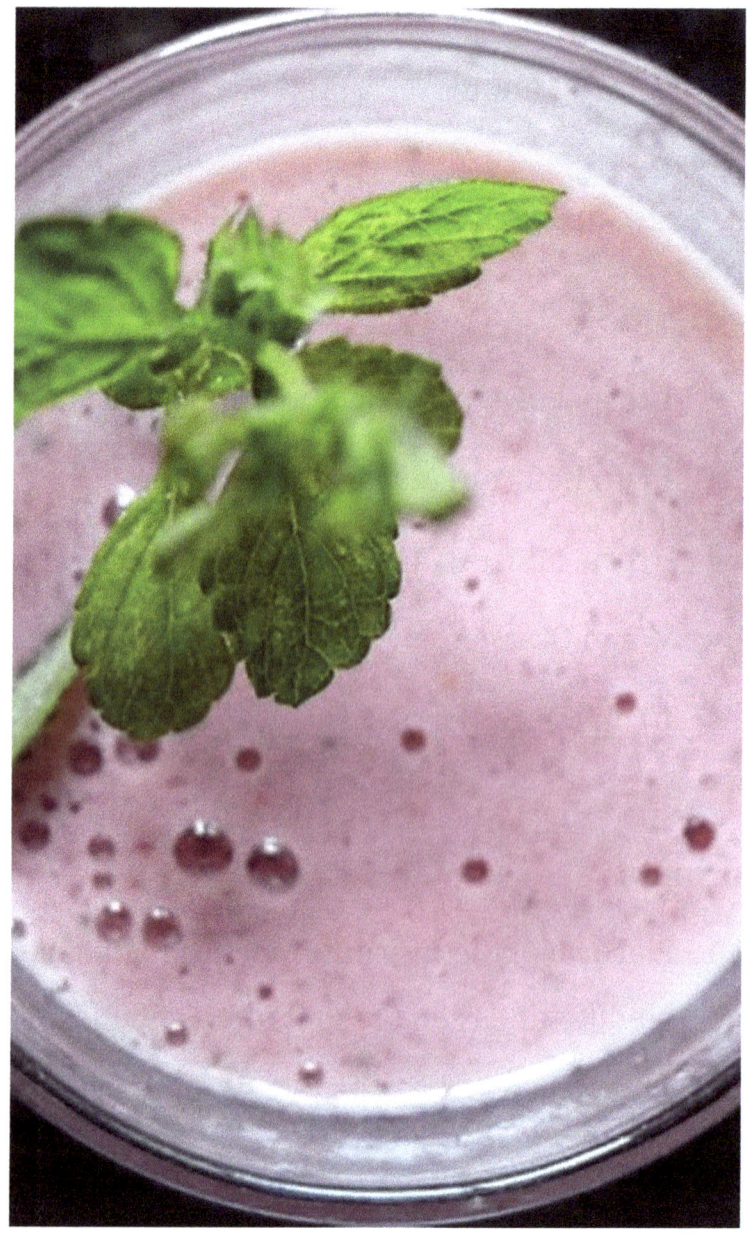

Greenie Smoothie

Preparation Time: *5 Minutes*

Cooking Time: 5 Minutes

Servings: *2*

Ingredients:

- 1 1/2 cup Water
- 1 tsp. Stevia
- 1 Green Apple, ripe
- 1 tsp. Stevia
- 1 Green Pear, chopped into chunks
- 1 Lime
- 2 cups Kale, fresh
- ¾ tsp. Cinnamon
- 12 Ice Cubes
- 20 Green Grapes
- 1/2 cup Mint, fresh

Directions:

1. Pour water, kale, and pear in a high-speed blender and blend them for 2 to 3 minutes until mixed.

2. Stir in all the remaining **Ingredients** into it and blend until it becomes smooth.

3. Transfer the smoothie to **Serving** glass.

Nutrition: Calories: 123Kcal; Carbohydrates: 27g; Proteins: 2g; Fat: 2g; Sodium: 30mg

Coconut Spinach Smoothie

Preparation Time: *5 Minutes*

Cooking Time: 5 Minutes

Servings: *2*

Ingredients:

- 1 ¼ cup Coconut Milk
- 2 Ice Cubes
- 2 tbsp. Chia Seeds
- 1 scoop of Protein Powder, preferably vanilla
- 1 cup Spin

Directions:

1. Pour coconut milk along with spinach, chia seeds, protein powder, and ice cubes in a high-speed blender.
2. Blend for 2 minutes to get a smooth and luscious smoothie.

3. Serve in a glass and enjoy it.

Nutrition: Calories: 251Kcal; Carbohydrates: 10.9g; Proteins: 20.3g; Fat: 15.1g; Sodium: 102mg

Oats Coffee Smoothie

Preparation Time: *5 Minutes*

Cooking Time: 5 Minutes

Servings: *2*

Ingredients:

- 1 cup Oats, uncooked & grounded
- 2 tbsp. Instant Coffee
- 3 cup Milk, skimmed
- 2 Banana, frozen & sliced into chunks
- 2 tbsp. Flax Seeds, grounded

Directions:

1. Place all of the **Ingredients** in a high-speed blender and blend for 2 minutes or until smooth and luscious.
2. Serve and enjoy.

Nutrition: Calories: 251Kcal; Carbohydrates: 10.9g; Proteins: 20.3g; Fat: 15.1g; Sodium: 102mg

Veggie Smoothie

Preparation Time: *5 Minutes*

<u>**Cooking Time**</u>: 5 Minutes

Servings: *1*

Ingredients:

- ¼ of 1 Red Bell Pepper, sliced
- 1/2 tbsp. Coconut Oil
- 1 cup Almond Milk, unsweetened
- ¼ tsp. Turmeric
- 4 Strawberries, chopped
- Pinch of Cinnamon
- 1/2 of 1 Banana, preferably frozen

Directions:

1. Combine all the **Ingredients** required to make the smoothie in a high-speed blender.

2. Blend for 3 minutes to get a smooth and silky mixture.
3. Serve and enjoy.

Nutrition: Calories: 169cal; Carbohydrates: 17g; Proteins: 2.3g; Fat: 9.8g; Sodium: 162mg

Avocado Smoothie

Preparation Time: *10 Minutes*

<u>Cooking Time</u>: 0 Minutes

Servings: *2*

Ingredients:

- 1 Avocado, ripe & pit removed
- 2 cups Baby Spinach
- 2 cups Water
- 1 cup Baby Kale
- 1 tbsp. Lemon Juice
- 2 sprigs of Mint
- 1/2 cup Ice Cubes

<u>Directions:</u>

1. Place all the Ingredients needed to make the smoothie in a high-speed blender then blend until smooth.

2. Transfer to a **Serving** glass and enjoy it.

Nutrition: Calories: 214cal; Carbohydrates: 15g; Proteins: 2g; Fat: 17g; Sodium: 25mg

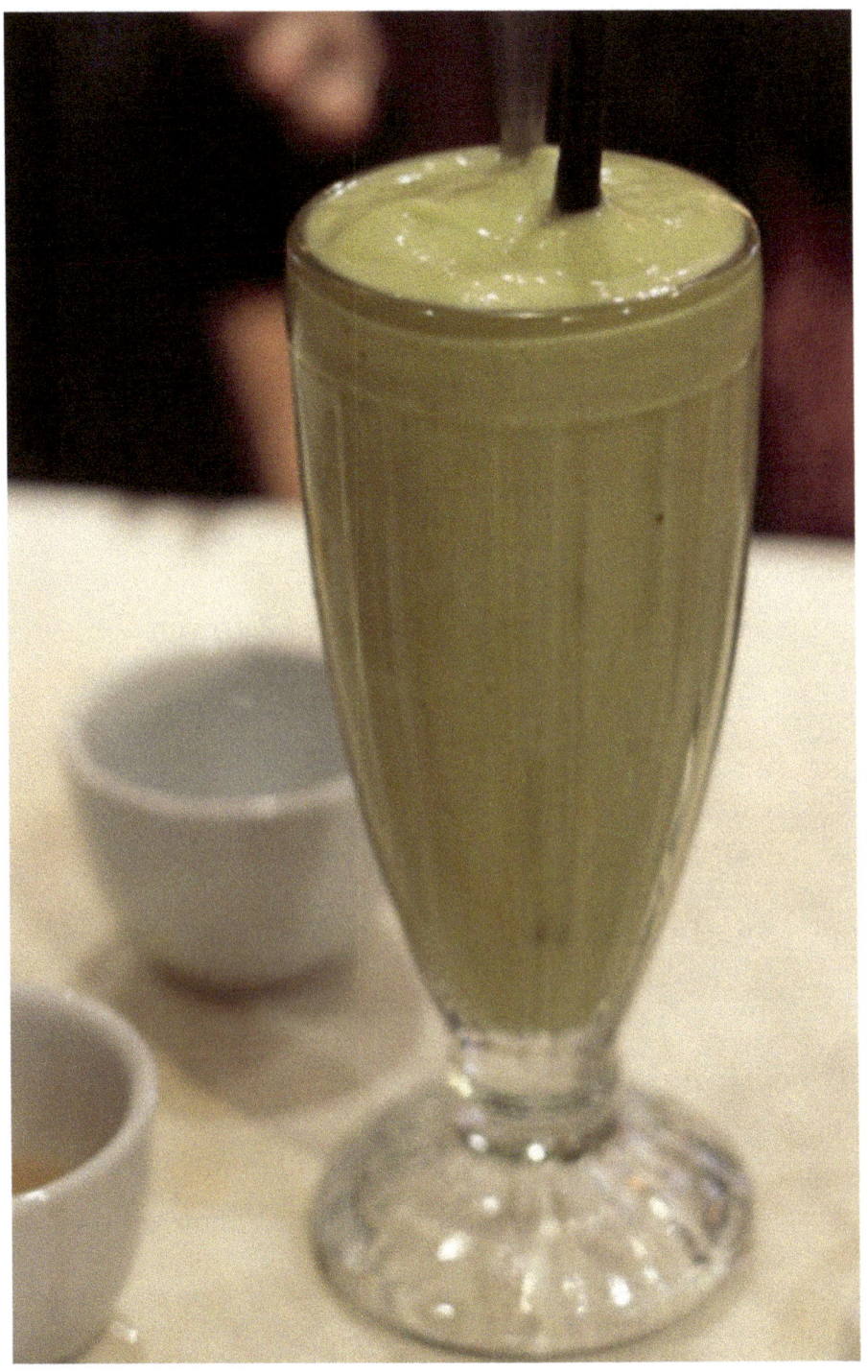

Orange Carrot Smoothie

Preparation Time: *5 Minutes*

<u>Cooking Time</u>: 0 Minutes

Servings: *1*

Ingredients:

- 1 1/2 cups Almond Milk
- ¼ cup Cauliflower, blanched & frozen
- 1 Orange
- 1 tbsp. Flax Seed
- 1/3 cup Carrot, grated
- 1 tsp. Vanilla Extract

Directions:

1. Mix all the Ingredients in a high-speed blender and blend for 2 minutes or until you get the desired consistency.
2. Transfer to a **Serving** glass and enjoy it.

Nutrition: Calories: 216cal; Carbohydrates: 10g; Proteins: 15g; Fat: 7g; Sodium: 25mg

Blackberry Smoothie

Preparation Time: 5 Minutes

Cooking Time: 0 Minutes

Servings: *1*

Ingredients:

- 1 1/2 cups Almond Milk
- ¼ cup Cauliflower, blanched & frozen
- 1 Orange
- 1 tbsp. Flax Seed
- 1/3 cup Carrot, grated
- 1 tsp. Vanilla Extract

Directions:

1. Place all the Ingredients needed to make the blackberry smoothie in a high-speed blender and blend for 2 minutes until you get a smooth mixture.

2. Transfer to a **Serving** glass and enjoy it.

Nutrition: Calories: 275cal; Carbohydrates: 9g; Proteins: 11g; Fat: 17g; Sodium: 73mg

Key Lime Pie Smoothie

Preparation Time: *5 Minutes*

<u>**Cooking Time**</u>: 0 Minutes

Servings: *1*

Ingredients:

- 1/2 cup Cottage Cheese
- 1 tbsp. Sweetener of your choice
- 1/2 cup Water
- 1/2 cup Spinach
- 1 tbsp. Lime Juice
- 1 cup Ice Cubes

Directions:

1. Spoon in the **Ingredients** to a high-speed blender and blend until silky smooth.
2. Transfer to a **Serving** glass and enjoy it.

Nutrition: Calories: 180cal; Carbohydrates: 7g; Proteins: 36g; Fat: 1g; Sodium: 35mg

Cinnamon Roll Smoothie

Preparation Time: *5 Minutes*

Cooking Time: 0 Minutes

Servings: *1*

Ingredients:

- 1 tsp. Flax Meal or oats, if preferred
- 1 cup Almond Milk
- 1/2 tsp. Cinnamon
- 2 tbsp. Protein Powder
- 1 cup Ice
- ¼ tsp. Vanilla Extract
- 4 tsp. Sweetener of your choice

Directions:

1. Pour the milk into the blender, followed by the protein powder, sweetener, flax meal, cinnamon, vanilla extract, and ice.

2. Blend for 40 seconds or until smooth.

3. Serve and enjoy.

Nutrition: Calories: 145cal; Carbohydrates: 1.6g; Proteins: 26.5g; Fat: 3.25g; Sodium: 30mg

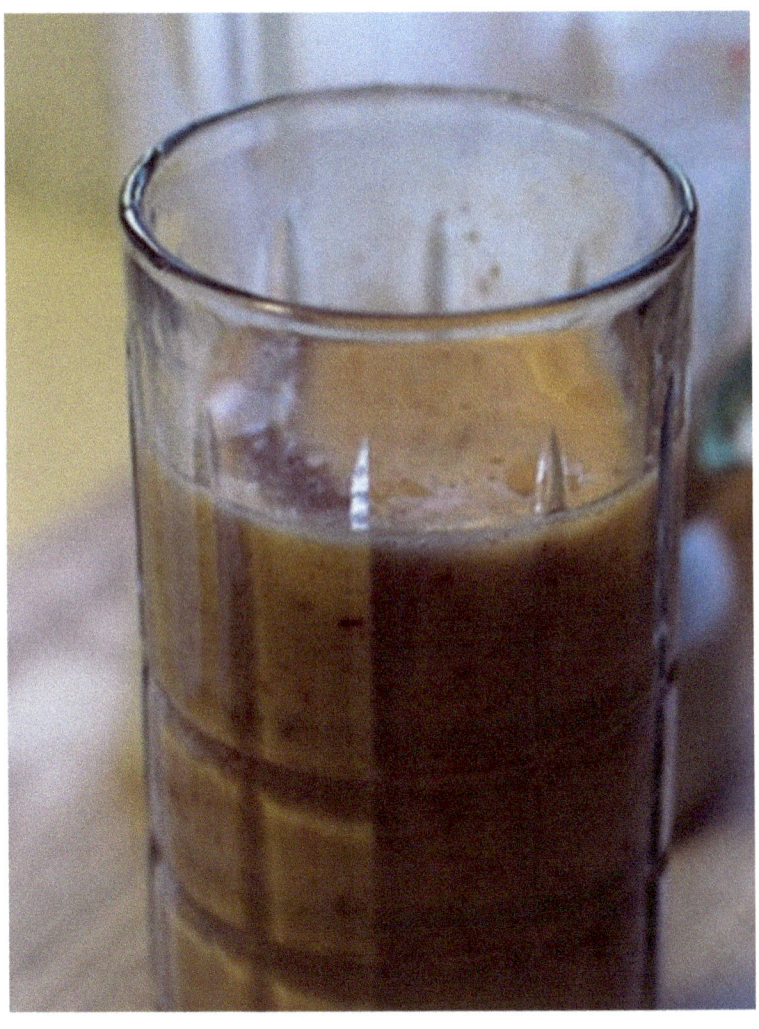

Strawberry Cheesecake Smoothie

Preparation Time: *5 Minutes*

Cooking Time: 0 Minutes

Servings: *1*

Ingredients:

- ¼ cup Soy Milk, unsweetened
- 1/2 cup Cottage Cheese, low-fat
- 1/2 tsp. Vanilla Extract
- 2 oz. Cream Cheese
- 1 cup Ice Cubes
- 1/2 cup Strawberries
- 4 tbsp. Low-carb Sweetener of your choice

Directions:

1. Add all the Ingredients for making the strawberry cheesecake smoothie to a high-

speed blender until you get the desired smooth consistency.

2. Serve and enjoy.

Nutrition: Calories: 347cal; Carbohydrates: 10.05g; Proteins: 17.5g; Fat: 24g; Sodium: 45mg

Peanut Butter Banana Smoothie

Preparation Time: *5 Minutes*

<u>**Cooking Time**</u>: 2 Minutes

Servings: *1*

Ingredients:

- ¼ cup Greek Yoghurt, plain
- 1/2 tbsp. Chia Seeds
- 1/2 cup Ice Cubes
- 1/2 of 1 Banana
- 1/2 cup Water
- 1 tbsp. Peanut Butter

<u>*Directions:*</u>

1. Place all the Ingredients needed to make the smoothie in a high-speed blender and blend to get a smooth and luscious mixture.

2. Transfer the smoothie to a **Serving** glass and enjoy it.

Nutrition: Calories: 202cal; Carbohydrates: 14g; Proteins: 10g; Fat: 9g; Sodium: 30mg

Avocado Turmeric Smoothie

Preparation Time: *5 Minutes*

<u>Cooking Time</u>: 2 Minutes

Servings: *1*

Ingredients:

- 1/2 of 1 Avocado
- 1 cup Ice, crushed
- ¾ cup Coconut Milk, full-fat
- 1 tsp. Lemon Juice
- ¼ cup Almond Milk
- 1/2 tsp. Turmeric
- 1 tsp. Ginger, freshly grated

Directions:

1. Place all the Ingredients excluding the crushed ice in a high-speed blender and blend for 2 to 3 minutes or until smooth.

2. Transfer to a **Serving** glass and enjoy it.

Nutrition: Calories: 232cal; Carbohydrates: 4.1g; Proteins: 1.7g; Fat: 22.4g; Sodium: 25mg

Lemon Blueberry Smoothie

Preparation Time: *5 Minutes*

Cooking Time: 2 Minutes

Servings: *2*

Ingredients:

- 1 tbsp. Lemon Juice
- 1 ¾ cup Coconut Milk, full-fat
- 1/2 tsp. Vanilla Extract
- 3 oz. Blueberries, frozen

Directions:

1. Combine coconut milk, blueberries, lemon juice, and vanilla extract in a high-speed blender.
2. Blend for 2 minutes for a smooth and luscious smoothie.
3. Serve and enjoy.

Nutrition: Calories: 417cal; Carbohydrates: 9g;Proteins: 4g; Fat: 43g; Sodium: 35mg

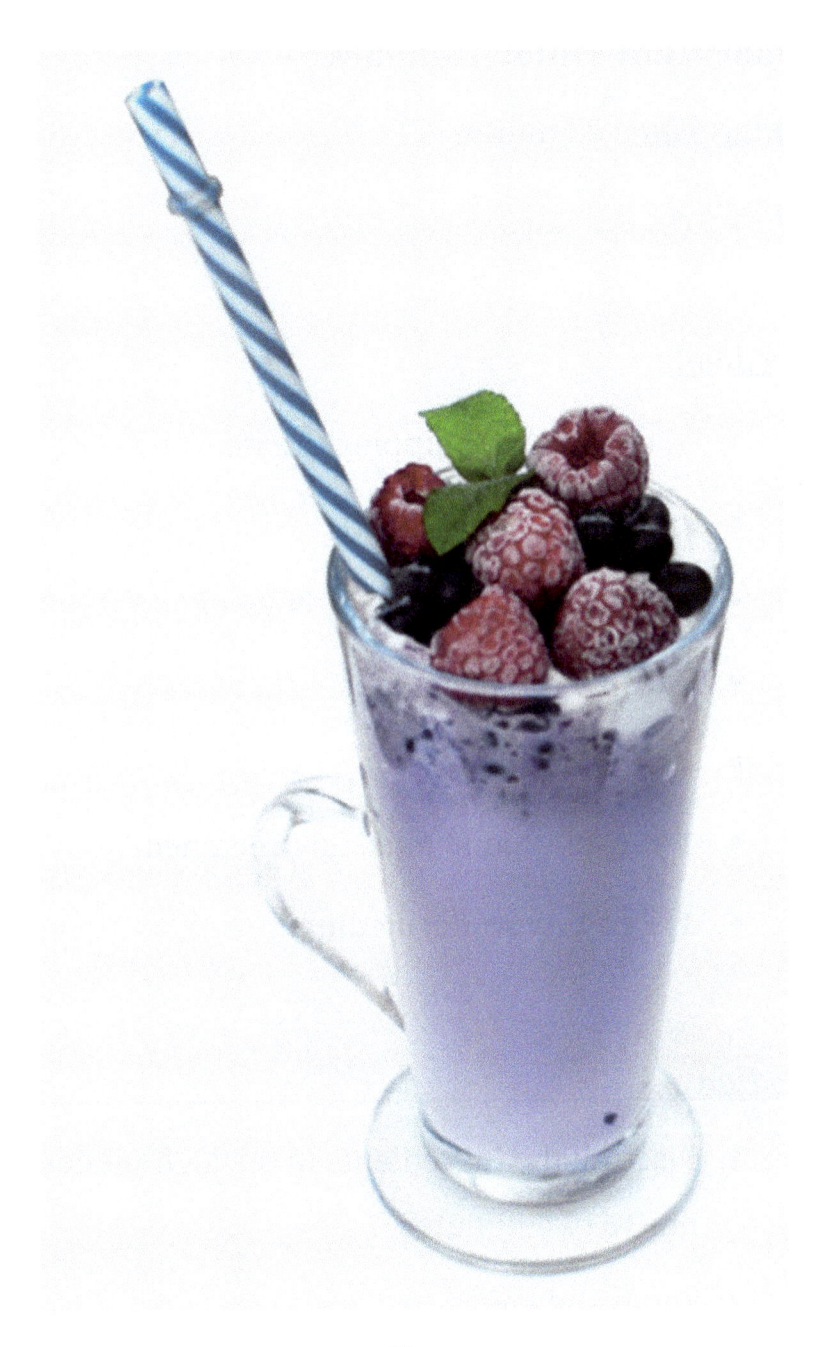

Matcha Green Smoothie

Preparation Time: *5 Minutes*

Cooking Time: 2 Minutes

Servings: *2*

Ingredients:

- ¼ cup Heavy Whipping Cream
- 1/2 tsp. Vanilla Extract
- 1 tsp. Matcha Green Tea Powder
- 2 tbsp. Protein Powder
- 1 tbsp. Hot Water
- 1 ¼ cup Almond Milk, unsweetened
- 1/2 of 1 Avocado, medium

Directions:

1. Place all the Ingredients in the high-blender for one to two minutes.
2. Serve and enjoy.

Nutrition: Calories: 229cal; Carbohydrates: 1.5g; Proteins: 14.1g; Fat: 43g; Sodium: 35mg

Blueberry Smoothie

Preparation Time: 10 minutes

Cooking Time: 0 minutes

Servings: *2*

Ingredients:

- 2 cups frozen blueberries
- 1 small banana
- 1½ cups unsweetened almond milk
- ¼ cup ice cubes

Directions:

1. Place all the Ingredients in a high-speed blender and pulse until creamy.
2. Pour the smoothie into two glasses and serve immediately.

Nutrition: Calories 158; Total Fat 3.3 g; Saturated Fat 0.3 g; Cholesterol 0 mg; Sodium 137 mg; Total Carbs 34 g; Fiber 5.6 g; Sugar 20.6 g; Protein 2.4 g

Beet & Strawberry Smoothie

Preparation Time: 10 minutes

Cooking Time: 0 minutes

Servings: *2*

Ingredients:

- 2 cups frozen strawberries, pitted and chopped
- 2/3 cup roasted and frozen beet, chopped
- 1 teaspoon fresh ginger, peeled and grated
- 1 teaspoon fresh turmeric, peeled and grated
- ½ cup fresh orange juice
- 1 cup unsweetened almond milk

Directions:

1. Place all the Ingredients in a high-speed blender and pulse until creamy.
2. Pour the smoothie into two glasses and serve immediately.

Nutrition: Calories 258; Total Fat 1.5 g; Saturated Fat 0.1 g; Cholesterol 0 mg; Sodium 134 mg; Total Carbs 26.7g; Fiber 4.9 g; Sugar 18.7 g; Protein 2.9 g

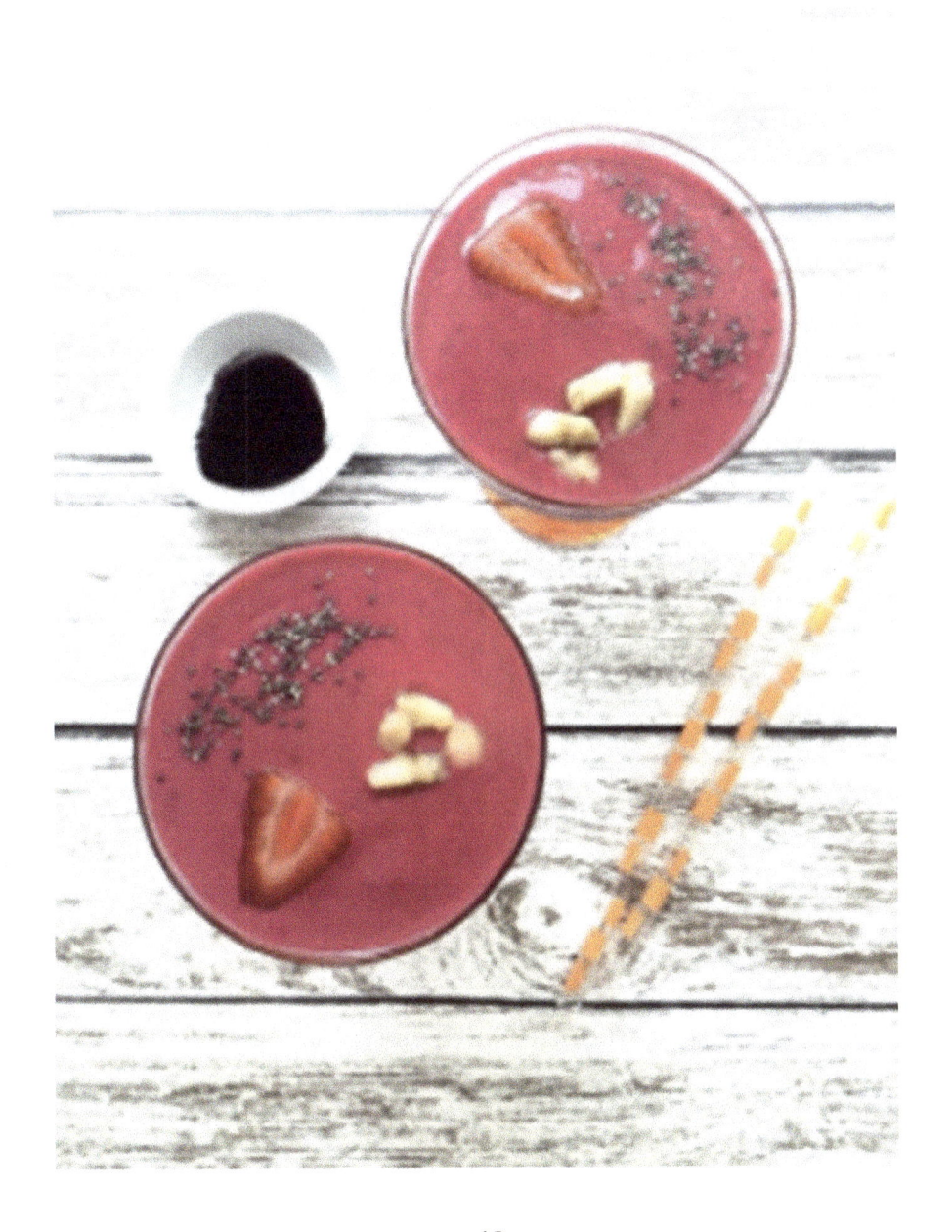

Kiwi Smoothie

Preparation Time: 10 minutes

Cooking Time: 0 minutes

Servings: *2*

Ingredients:

- 4 kiwis
- 2 small bananas, peeled
- 1½ cups unsweetened almond milk
- 1-2 drops liquid stevia
- ¼ cup ice cubes

Directions:

1. Place all the **Ingredients** in a high-speed blender and pulse until creamy.
2. Pour the smoothie into two glasses and serve immediately.

Nutrition: Calories 228 Total Fat; 3.8 g Saturated Fat 0.4 g; Cholesterol 0 mg; Sodium 141 mg; Total Carbs 50.7 g; Fiber 8.4 g; Sugar 28.1 g; Protein 3.8 g

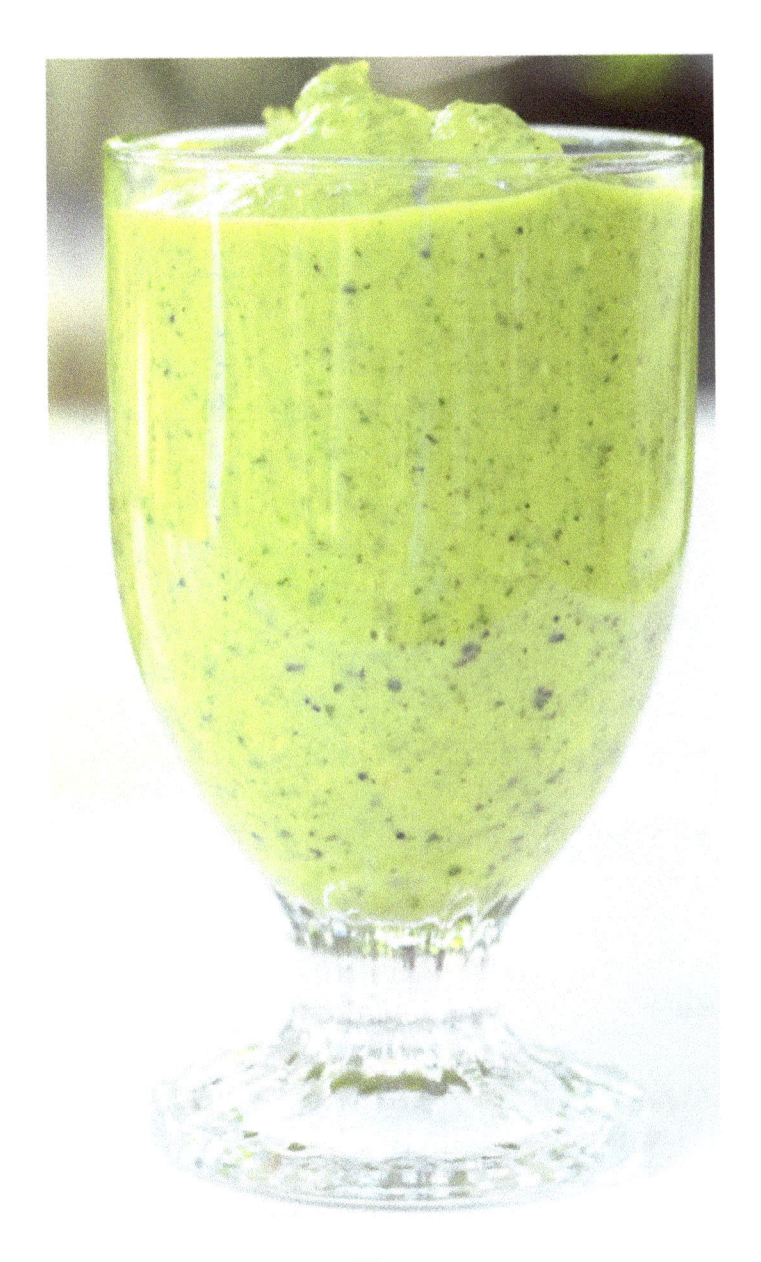

Pineapple & Carrot Smoothie

Preparation Time: 10 minutes

***Cooking Time*:** 0 minutes

Servings: *2*

Ingredients:

- 1 cup frozen pineapple
- 1 large ripe banana, peeled and sliced
- ½ tablespoon fresh ginger, peeled and chopped
- ¼ teaspoon ground turmeric
- 1 cup unsweetened almond milk
- ½ cup fresh carrot juice
- 1 tablespoon fresh lemon juice

Directions:

1. Place all the **Ingredients** in a high-speed blender and pulse until creamy.

2. Pour the smoothie into two glasses and serve immediately.

Nutrition: Calories 132; Total Fat 2.2 g; Saturated Fat 0.3 g; Cholesterol 0 mg; Sodium 113 mg; Total Carbs 629.3 g; Fiber 4.1 g; Sugar 16.9 g; Protein 2 g;

Oats & Orange Smoothie

Preparation Time: 10 minutes

Cooking Time: 0 minutes

Servings: *4*

Ingredients:

- 2/3 cup rolled oats
- 2 oranges, peeled, seeded, and sectioned
- 2 large bananas, peeled and sliced
- 2 cups unsweetened almond milk
- 1 cup ice cubes, crushed

Directions:

1. Place all the **Ingredients** in a high-speed blender and pulse until creamy.
2. Pour the smoothie into four glasses and serve immediately.

Nutrition: Calories 175; Total Fat 3 g; Saturated Fat 0.4 g; Cholesterol 0 mg; Sodium 93 mg; Total Carbs 36.6 g; Fiber 5.9 g, Sugar 17.1 g, Protein 3.9 g;

Pumpkin Smoothie

Preparation Time: 10 minutes

Cooking Time: 0 minutes

Servings: *2*

Ingredients:

- 1 cup homemade pumpkin puree
- 1 medium banana, peeled and sliced
- 1 tablespoon maple syrup
- 1 teaspoon ground flaxseeds
- ½ teaspoon ground cinnamon
- ¼ teaspoon ground ginger
- 1½ cups unsweetened almond milk
- ¼ cup ice cubes

Directions:

1. Place all the **Ingredients** in a high-speed blender and pulse until creamy.
2. Pour the smoothie into two glasses and serve immediately.

Nutrition: Calories 159; Total Fat 3.6 g; Saturated Fat 0.5 g; Cholesterol 0 mg; Sodium 143 mg; Total Carbs 32.6 g; Fiber 6.5 g, Sugar 17.3 g; Protein 3 g

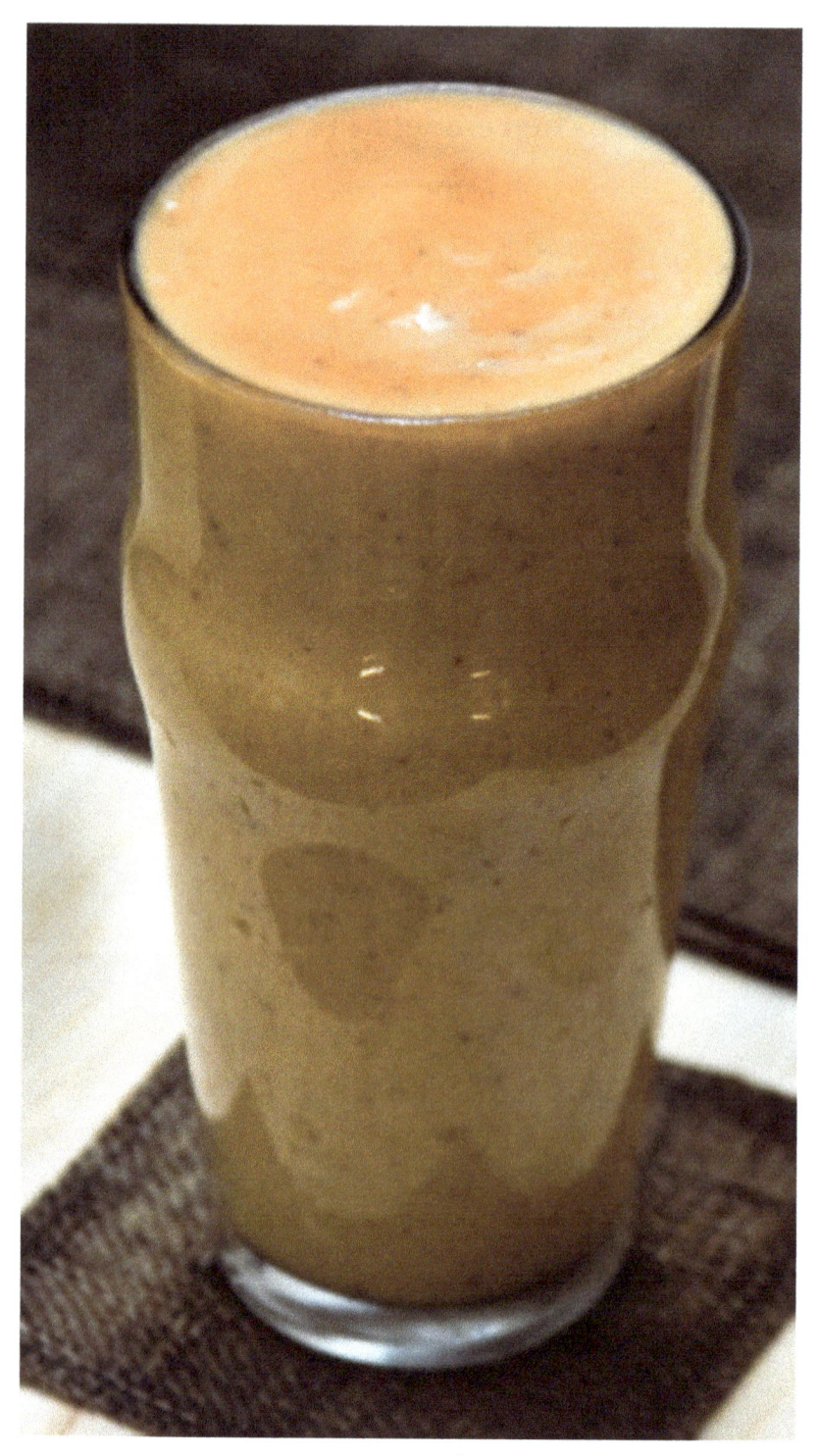

Red Veggie & Fruit Smoothie

Preparation Time: 10 minutes

Cooking Time: 0 minutes

Servings: 2

Ingredients:

- ½ cup fresh raspberries
- ½ cup fresh strawberries
- ½ red bell pepper, seeded and chopped
- ½ cup red cabbage, chopped
- 1 small tomato
- 1 cup water
- ½ cup ice cubes

Directions:

1. Place all the **Ingredients** in a high-speed blender and pulse until creamy.

2. Pour the smoothie into two glasses and serve immediately.

Nutrition: Calories 39; Cholesterol 0 mg; Saturated Fat 0 g; Sodium 10 mg; Total Carbs 8.9 g; Fiber 3.5 g; Sugar 4.8 g; Protein 1.3 g, Total Fat 0.4 g

Kale Smoothie

Preparation Time: 10 minutes

Cooking Time: 0 minutes

Servings: 2

Ingredients:

- 3 stalks fresh kale, trimmed and chopped
- 1-2 celery stalks, chopped
- ½ avocado, peeled, pitted, and chopped
- ½-inch piece ginger root, chopped
- ½-inch piece turmeric root, chopped
- 2 cups coconut milk

Directions:

1. Place all the **Ingredients** in a high-speed blender and pulse until creamy.
2. Pour the smoothie into two glasses and serve immediately.

Nutrition: Calories 248; Total Fat 21.8 g; Saturated Fat 12 g; Cholesterol 0 mg; Sodium 59 mg; Total Carbs 11.3 g; Fiber 4.2 g; Sugar 0.5 g, Protein 3.5 g

Green Tofu Smoothie

Preparation Time: 10 minutes

Cooking Time: 0 minutes

Servings: 2

Ingredients:

- 1½ cups cucumber, peeled and chopped roughly
- 3 cups fresh baby spinach
- 2 cups frozen broccoli
- ½ cup silken tofu, drained and pressed
- 1 tablespoon fresh lime juice
- 4-5 drops liquid stevia
- 1 cup unsweetened almond milk
- ½ cup ice, crushed

Directions:

1. Place all the **Ingredients** in a high-speed blender and pulse until creamy.
2. Pour the smoothie into two glasses and serve immediately.

Nutrition: Calories 118; Total Fat 15 g; Saturated Fat 0.8 g; Cholesterol 0 mg; Sodium 165 mg; Total Carbs 12.6 g; Fiber 4.8 g; Sugar 3.4 g; Protein 10 g

Grape & Swiss Chard Smoothie

Preparation Time: 10 minutes

Cooking Time: 0 minutes

Servings: 2

Ingredients:

- 2 cups seedless green grapes
- 2 cups fresh Swiss chard, trimmed and chopped
- 2 tablespoons maple syrup
- 1 teaspoon fresh lemon juice
- 1½ cups water
- 4 ice cubes

Directions:

1. Place all the **Ingredients** in a high-speed blender and pulse until creamy.

2. Pour the smoothie into two glasses and serve immediately.

Nutrition: Calories 176; Total Fat 0.2 g; Saturated Fat 0 g; Cholesterol 0 mg; Sodium 83 mg; Total Carbs 44.9 g; Fiber 1.7 g; Sugar 37.9 g; Protein 0.7 g

Matcha Smoothie

Preparation Time: 10 minutes

Cooking Time: *0 minutes*

Servings: *2*

Ingredients:

- 2 tablespoons chia seeds
- 2 teaspoons matcha green tea powder
- ½ teaspoon fresh lemon juice
- ½ teaspoon xanthan gum
- 8-10 drops liquid stevia
- 4 tablespoons coconut cream
- 1½ cups unsweetened almond milk
- ¼ cup ice cubes

Directions:

1. Place all the **Ingredients** in a high-speed blender and pulse until creamy.

2. Pour the smoothie into two glasses and serve immediately.

Nutrition: Calories 132; Total Fat 12.3 g; Saturated Fat 6.8 g; Cholesterol 0 mg; Sodium 15 mg; Total Carbs 7 g; Fiber 4.8 g; Sugar 1 g; Protein 3 g

Banana Smoothie

Preparation Time: 10 minutes

Cooking Time: *0 minutes*

Servings: *2*

Ingredients:

- 2 cups chilled unsweetened almond milk
- 1 large frozen banana, peeled and sliced
- 1 tablespoon almonds, chopped
- 1 teaspoon organic vanilla extract

Directions:

1. Place all the **Ingredients** in a high-speed blender and pulse until creamy.
2. Pour the smoothie into two glasses and serve immediately.

Nutrition: Calories 124; Total Fat 5.2 g; Saturated Fat 0.5 g; Cholesterol 0 mg; Sodium 181 mg; Total Carbs 18.4 g; Fiber 3.1 g; Sugar 8.7 g; Protein 2.4 g

Strawberry Smoothie

Preparation Time: 10 minutes

Cooking Time: *0 minutes*

Servings: 2

Ingredients:

- 2 cups chilled unsweetened almond milk
- 1½ cups frozen strawberries
- 1 banana, peeled and sliced
- ¼ teaspoon organic vanilla extract

Directions:

1. Add all the **Ingredients** in a high-speed blender and pulse until smooth.
2. Pour the smoothie into two glasses and serve immediately.

Nutrition: Calories 131; Total Fat 3.7 g; Saturated Fat 0.4 g; Cholesterol 0 mg; Sodium 181 mg; Total Carbs 25.3 g; Fiber 4.8 g; Sugar 14 g; Protein 1.6 g

Raspberry & Tofu Smoothie

Preparation Time: 15 minutes

Cooking Time: *0 minutes*

Servings: *2*

Ingredients:

- 1½ cups fresh raspberries
- 6 ounces firm silken tofu, drained
- 1/8 teaspoon coconut extract
- 1 teaspoon powdered stevia
- 1½ cups unsweetened almond milk
- ¼ cup ice cubes, crushed

Directions:

1. Add all the **Ingredients** in a high-speed blender and pulse until smooth.
2. Pour the smoothie into two glasses and serve immediately.

Nutrition: Calories 131; Total Fat 5.5 g; Saturated Fat 0.6 g; Cholesterol 0 mg; Sodium 167 mg; Total Carbs 14.6 g; Fiber 6.8 g; Sugar 5.2 g, Protein 7.7 g

Mango Smoothie

Preparation Time: 10 minutes

Cooking Time: *0 minutes*

Servings: *2*

Ingredients:

- 2 cups frozen mango, peeled, pitted and chopped
- ¼ cup almond butter
- Pinch of ground turmeric
- 2 tablespoons fresh lemon juice
- 1¼ cups unsweetened almond milk
- ¼ cup ice cubes

Directions:

1. Add all the **Ingredients** in a high-speed blender and pulse until smooth.

2. Pour the smoothie into two glasses and serve immediately.

Nutrition: Calories 140; Total Fat 4.1 g; Saturated Fat 0.6 g; Cholesterol 0 mg; Sodium 118 mg; Total Carbs 26.8 g; Fiber 3.6 g; Sugar 23 g; Protein 2.5 g

Pineapple Smoothie

Preparation Time: 10 minutes

Cooking Time: *0 minutes*

Servings: *2*

Ingredients:

- 2 cups pineapple, chopped
- ½ teaspoon fresh ginger, peeled and chopped
- ½ teaspoon ground turmeric
- 1 teaspoon natural immune support supplement *
- 1 teaspoon chia seeds
- 1½ cups cold green tea
- ½ cup ice, crushed

Directions:

1. Add all the **Ingredients** in a high-speed blender and pulse until smooth.

2. Pour the smoothie into two glasses and serve immediately.

Nutrition: Calories 152; Total Fat 1 g; Saturated Fat 0 g; Cholesterol 0 mg; Sodium 9 mg; Total Carbs 30 g; Fiber 3.5 g; Sugar 29.8 g; Protein 1.5 g

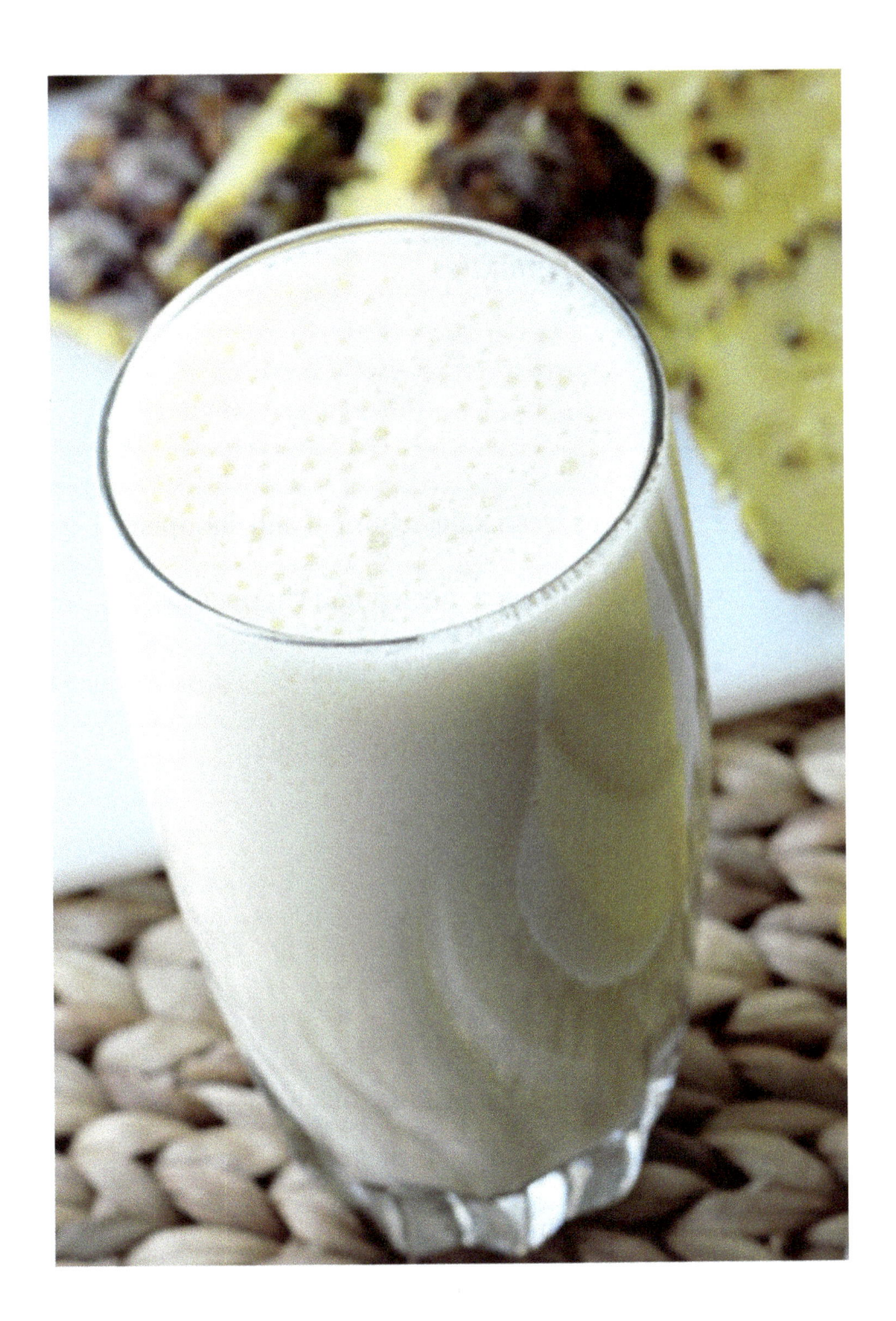

Kale & Pineapple Smoothie

Preparation Time: 15 minutes

Cooking Time: *0 minutes*

Servings: *2*

Ingredients:

- 1½ cups fresh kale, trimmed and chopped
- 1 frozen banana, peeled and chopped
- ½ cup fresh pineapple chunks
- 1 cup unsweetened coconut milk
- ½ cup fresh orange juice
- ½ cup ice

Directions:

1. Add all the **Ingredients** in a high-speed blender and pulse until smooth.
2. Pour the smoothie into two glasses and serve immediately.

Nutrition: Calories 148; Total Fat 2.4 g; Saturated Fat 2.1 g; Cholesterol 0 mg; Sodium 23 mg; Total Carbs 31.6 g; Fiber 3.5 g; Sugar 16.5 g; Protein 2.8 g

Green Veggies Smoothie

Preparation Time: 15 minutes

Cooking Time: *0 minutes*

Servings: *2*

Ingredients:

- 1 medium avocado, peeled, pitted, and chopped
- 1 large cucumber, peeled and chopped
- 2 fresh tomatoes, chopped
- 1 small green bell pepper, seeded and chopped
- 1 cup fresh spinach, torn
- 2 tablespoons fresh lime juice
- 2 tablespoons homemade vegetable broth
- 1 cup alkaline water

Directions:

1. Add all the **Ingredients** in a high-speed blender and pulse until smooth.
2. Pour the smoothie into glasses and serve immediately.

Nutrition: Calories 275; Total Fat 20.3 g; Saturated Fat 4.2 g; Cholesterol 0 mg; Sodium 76 mg; Total Carbs 24.1 g; Fiber 10.1 g; Sugar 9.3 g; Protein 5.3 g

Avocado & Spinach Smoothie

Preparation Time: 10 minutes

Cooking Time: *0 minutes*

Servings: *2*

Ingredients:

- 2 cups fresh baby spinach
- ½ avocado, peeled, pitted, and chopped
- 4-6 drops liquid stevia
- ½ teaspoon ground cinnamon
- 1 tablespoon hemp seeds
- 2 cups chilled alkaline water

Directions:

1. Add all the **Ingredients** in a high-speed blender and pulse until smooth.
2. Pour the smoothie into two glasses and serve immediately.

Nutrition: Calories 132; Total Fat 11.7 g; Saturated Fat 2.2 g; Cholesterol 0 mg; Sodium 27 mg; Total Carbs 6.1 g; Fiber 4.5 g; Sugar 0.4 g; Protein 3.1 g

Raisins – Plume Smoothie (RPS)

<u>Preparation Time:</u> 10 minutes

<u>Cooking Time</u>: 0 minutes

Servings: *1*

Ingredients:

- 1 Teaspoon Raisins
- 2 Sweet Cherry
- 1 Skinned Black Plume
- 1 Cup Dr. Sebi's Stomach Calming Herbal Tea/ Cuachalate back powder,
- ¼ Coconut Water

Directions:

1. Flash 1 teaspoon of Raisin in warm water for 5 seconds and drain the water completely.
2. Rinse, cube Sweet Cherry and skinned black Plum

3. Get 1 cup of water boiled; put ¾ Dr. Sebi's Stomach Calming Herbal Tea for 10 – 15minutes.

4. If you are unable to get Dr. Sebi's Stomach Calming Herbal tea, you can alternatively, cook 1 teaspoon of powdered Cuachalate with 1 cup of water for 5 – 10 minutes, remove the extract and allow it to cool.

5. Pour all the ARPS items inside a blender and blend till you achieve a homogenous smoothie.

6. It is now okay, for you to enjoy the inevitable detox smoothie.

Nutrition: Calories: 150; Fat: 1.2 g; Carbohydrates: 79 g; Protein: 3.1 g

Nori Clove Smoothies (NCS)

Preparation Time: 10 minutes

Cooking Time: 0 minutes

Servings: *1*

Ingredients:

- ¼ Cup Fresh Nori
- 1 Cup Cubed Banana
- 1 Teaspoon Diced Onion or ¼ Teaspoon Powdered Onion
- ½ Teaspoon Clove
- 1 Cup Dr. Sebi Energy Booster
- 1 Tablespoon Agave Syrup

Directions:

1. Rinse ANCS Items with clean water.
2. Finely chop the onion to take one teaspoon and cut fresh Nori

3. Boil 1½ teaspoon with 2 cups of water, remove the particle, allow to cool, measure 1 cup of the tea extract

4. Pour all the items inside a blender with the tea extract and blend to achieve homogenous smoothies.

5. Transfer into a clean cup and have a nice time with a lovely body detox and energizer.

Nutrition: Calories: 78; Fat: 2.3 g; Carbohydrates: 5 g; Protein: 6 g

Brazil Lettuce Smoothies (BLS)

Preparation Time: 10 minutes

Cooking Time: 0 minutes

Servings: *1*

Ingredients:

- 1 Cup Raspberries
- ½ Handful Romaine Lettuce
- ½ Cup Homemade Walnut Milk
- 2 Brazil Nuts
- ½ Large Grape with Seed
- 1 Cup Soft jelly Coconut Water
- Date Sugar to Taste

Directions:

1. In a clean bowl rinse, the vegetable with clean water.

2. Chop the Romaine Lettuce and cubed Raspberries and add other items into the blender and blend to achieve homogenous smoothies.
3. Serve your delicious medicinal detox.

Nutrition: Calories: 168; Fat: 4.5 g; Carbohydrates: 31.3 g; Sugar: 19.2 g; Protein: 3.6 g

Apple – Banana Smoothie (Abs)

Preparation Time: 10 minutes

Cooking Time: 0 minutes

Servings: *1*

Ingredients:

- I Cup Cubed Apple
- ½ Burro Banana
- ½ Cup Cubed Mango
- ½ Cup Cubed Watermelon
- ½ Teaspoon Powdered Onion
- 3 Tablespoon Key Lime Juice
- Date Sugar to Taste (If you like)

Directions:

1. In a clean bowl rinse, the vegetable with clean water.

2. Cubed Banana, Apple, Mango, Watermelon and add other items into the blender and blend to achieve homogenous smoothies.

3. Serve your delicious medicinal detox.

4. Alternatively, you can add one tablespoon of finely dices raw red Onion if powdered Onion is not available.

Nutrition: Calories: 99; Fat: 0.3g; Carbohydrates: 23 grams; Protein: 1.1 g

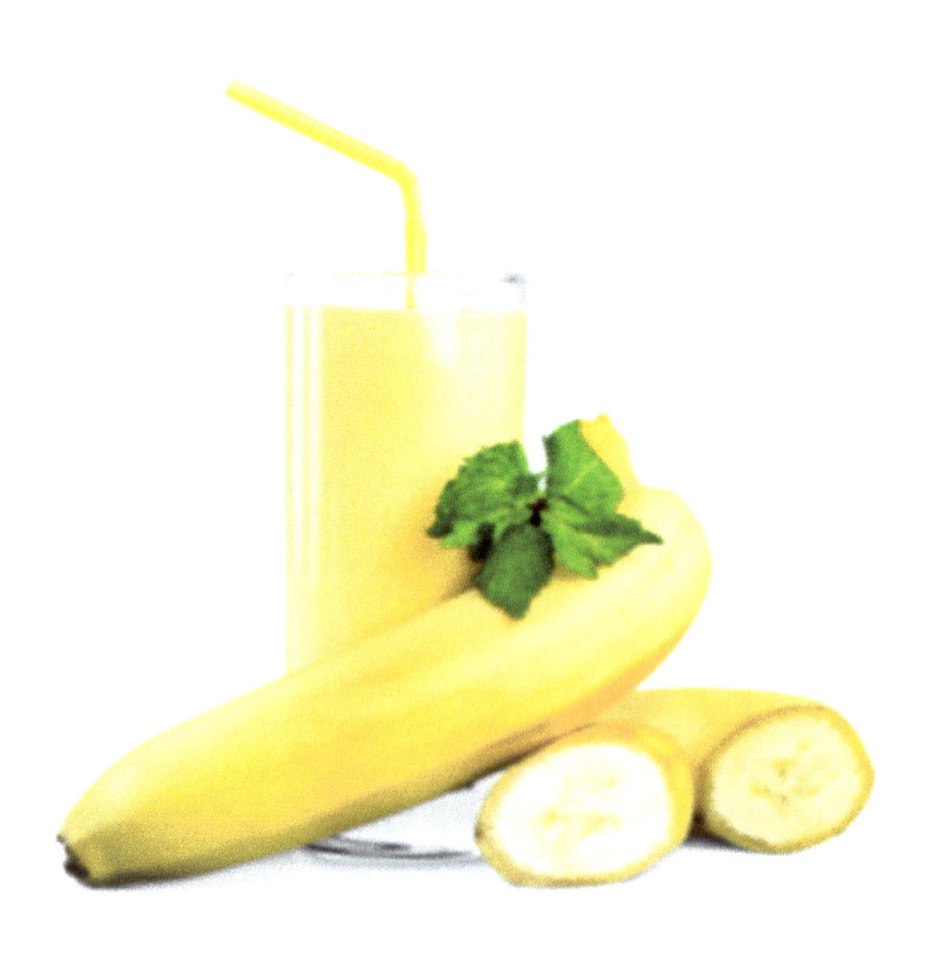

Ginger – Pear Smoothie (GPS)

Preparation Time: 10 minutes

Cooking Time: 0 minutes

Servings: *1*

Ingredients:

- 1 Big Pear with Seed and Cured
- ½ Avocado
- ¼ Handful Watercress
- ½ Sour Orange
- ½ Cup Ginger Tea
- ½ Cup Coconut Water
- ¼ Cup Spring Water
- 2 Tablespoon Agave Syrup
- Date Sugar to satisfaction

Directions:

1. Firstly boil 1 cup of Ginger Tea, cover the cup and allow it cool to room temperature.

2. Pour all the AGPS Items into your clean blender and homogenize them to smooth fluid.

3. You have just prepared yourself a wonderful Detox Romaine Smoothie.

Nutrition: Calories: 101; Protein: 1 g; Carbs: 27 g; Fiber: 6 g

Cantaloupe – Amaranth Smoothie (CAS)

Preparation Time: 10 minutes

Cooking Time: 0 minutes

Servings: *1*

Ingredients:

- ½ Cup Cubed Cantaloupe
- ¼ Handful Green Amaranth
- ½ Cup Homemade Hemp Milk
- ¼ Teaspoon Dr. Sebi's Bromide Plus Powder
- 1 Cup Coconut Water
- 1 Teaspoon Agave Syrup

Directions:

1. You will have to rinse all the ACAS items with clean water.

2. Chop green Amaranth, cubed Cantaloupe, transfer all into a blender and blend to achieve homogenous smoothie.

3. Pour into a clean cup; add Agave syrup and homemade Hemp Milk.

4. Stir them together and drink.

Nutrition: Calories: 55; Fiber: 1.5 g; Carbohydrates: 8 mg

Garbanzo Squash Smoothie (GSS)

Preparation Time: 10 minutes

Cooking Time: 0 minutes

Servings: 1

Ingredients:

- 1 Large Cubed Apple
- 1 Fresh Tomatoes
- 1 Tablespoon Finely Chopped Fresh Onion or ¼ Teaspoon Powdered Onion
- ¼ Cup Boiled Garbanzo Bean
- ½ Cup Coconut Milk
- ¼ Cubed Mexican Squash Chayote
- 1 Cup Energy Booster Tea

Directions:

1. You will need to rinse the AGSS items with clean water.

2. Boil 1½ Dr. Sebi's Energy Booster Tea with 2 cups of clean water. Filter the extract, measure 1 cup and allow it to cool.

3. Cook Garbanzo Bean, drain the water and allow it to cool.

4. Pour all the AGSS items into a high-speed blender and blend to achieve homogenous smoothie.

5. You may add Date Sugar.

6. Serve your amazing smoothie and drink.

Nutrition: Calories: 82; Carbs: 22 g; Protein: 2 g; Fiber: 7 g

Strawberry – Orange Smoothies (SOS)

Preparation Time: 10 minutes

Cooking Time: 0 minutes

Servings: *1*

Ingredients:

- 1 Cup Diced Strawberries
- 1 Removed Back of Seville Orange
- ¼ Cup Cubed Cucumber
- ¼ Cup Romaine Lettuce
- ½ Kelp
- ½ Burro Banana
- 1 Cup Soft Jelly Coconut Water
- ½ Cup Water
- Date Sugar.

Directions:

1. Use clean water to rinse all the vegetable items of ASOS into a clean bowl.

2. Chop Romaine Lettuce; dice Strawberry, Cucumber, and Banana; remove the back of Seville Orange and divide into four.

3. Transfer all the ASOS items inside a clean blender and blend to achieve a homogenous smoothie.

4. Pour into a clean big cup and fortify your body with a palatable detox.

Nutrition: Calories 298; Calories from Fat 9; Fat 1g; Cholesterol 2mg; Sodium 73mg; Potassium 998mg; Carbohydrates 68g; Fiber 7g; Sugar 50g

Tamarind – Pear Smoothie (TPS)

Preparation Time: 10 minutes

Cooking Time: 0 minutes

Servings: *1*

Ingredients:

- ½ Burro Banana
- ½ Cup Watermelon
- 1 Raspberries
- 1 Prickly Pear
- 1 Grape with Seed
- 3 Tamarind
- ½ Medium Cucumber
- 1 Cup Coconut Water
- ½ Cup Distilled Water

Directions:

1. Use clean water to rinse all the ATPS items.

2. Remove the pod of Tamarind and collect the edible part around the seed into a container.

3. If you must use the seeds then you have to boil the seed for 15mins and add to the Tamarind edible part in the container.

4. Cubed all other vegetable fruits and transfer all the items into a high-speed blender and blend to achieve homogenous smoothie.

Nutrition: Calories: 199; Carbohydrates: 47 g; Fat: 1g; Protein: 6g

Currant Elderberry Smoothie (CES)

Preparation Time: 10 minutes

Cooking Time: 0 minutes

Servings: *1*

Ingredients:

- ¼ Cup Cubed Elderberry
- 1 Sour Cherry
- 2 Currant
- 1 Cubed Burro Banana
- 1 Fig
- 1Cup 4 Bay Leaves Tea
- 1 Cup Energy Booster Tea
- Date Sugar to your satisfaction

Directions:

1. Use clean water to rinse all the ACES items

2. Initially boil ¾ Teaspoon of Energy Booster Tea with 2 cups of water on a heat source and allow boiling for 10 minutes.
3. Add 4 Bay leaves and boil together for another 4minutes.
4. Drain the Tea extract into a clean big cup and allow it to cool.
5. Transfer all the items into a high-speed blender and blend till you achieve a homogenous smoothie.
6. Pour the palatable medicinal smoothie into a clean cup and drink.

Nutrition: Calories: 63; Fat: 0.22g; Sodium: 1.1mg; Carbohydrates: 15.5g; Fiber: 4.8g; Sugars: 8.25g; Protein: 1.6g

Sweet Dream Strawberry Smoothie

Preparation Time: 1-5 minutes

Cooking Time: 0

Servings: 1

Ingredients:

- 5 Strawberries
- 3 Dates – Pits eliminated
- 2 Burro Bananas or small bananas
- Spring Water for 32 fluid ounces of smoothie

Directions:

1. Strip off skin of the bananas.
2. Wash the dates and strawberries.
3. Include bananas, dates, and strawberries to a blender container.
4. Include a couple of water and blend.

5. Keep on including adequate water to persuade up to be 32 oz. of smoothie.

Nutrition: Calories: 282; Fat: 11g; Carbohydrates: 4g; Protein: 7g

Lightning Source UK Ltd.
Milton Keynes UK
UKHW020815180621
385734UK00005B/55